Contents

What is the GAPS Diet?

The GAPS diet is a comprehensive healing protocol developed by Dr. Natasha Campbell-McBride, a neurologist and nutritionist who specializes in healing of issues like autism spectrum disorders, ADD/ADHD, dyspraxia, dyslexia and schizophrenia by treating the root cause of many of these disorders: compromised gut health.

While it may seem strange or even unbelievable that neurological disorders like autism can be mitigated or even addressed through dietary changes, families that have been dissatisfied by currently available treatments have flocked to the GAPS diet, and many have experienced recovery.

About 10% of Nourished Kitchen readers adhere to the GAPS diet (that's about twice the number of both vegan and vegetarian readers). Mothers and fathers have seen autistic children begin to lose symptoms, find relief from painful gastrointestinal upset and regain the ability to express emotion after adhering to the GAPS diet. People suffering from food intolerances and sensitivities have seen recovery. Recovery takes time, and the GAPS diet doesn't work overnight. Indeed, GAPS is best referred to as a healing protocol as it involves both comprehensive detoxification coupled with dietary changes and supplementation.

GAPS begins first with an introduction diet (though many people, to ease their transition begin first by incorporating the full GAPS diet and return to the introduction phases at a future date when they feel more confident in their transition). In the introduction diet offers about six stages before the full GAPS diet can be resumed, with the beginning stages allowing little more than broth, good quality fat, easily digested vegetables, boiled meats and the juice of fermented vegetables. You eat lots of soups on the GAPS diet.

Once symptoms no longer appear, additional foods like fruit, raw vegetables and their juices, nuts and nut flours are slowly added until you've reached the full GAPS diet which allows most wholesome foods, but still excludes grains, starchy tubers, sugars (except for honey) and other foods that can potentially damage an already compromised gut.

Theory behind how the GAPS diet works

The concept of GAPS and the GAPS diet were created by Natasha Campbell-McBride, MD, a physician who spent her career working as a neurologist and later a nutritionist in her own clinic.

According to Campbell-McBride's theory, large growths of bad bacteria in the gut give off toxic substances like acetaldehyde and clostridial neurotoxins when digesting food. Her theory, which is unproven, is that these toxins then enter the bloodstream where they can harm your immune system, organs, and cause psychiatric and neurological problems.

The GAPS diet claims to prevent this by promoting "good" bacterial growth in the gut and eliminating high-fiber, inflammatory foods.

What You Need to Know

Dr. Campbell-McBride recommends that people hoping to achieve results from the GAPS diet start with the introductory phase and stay on it (working through its six stages) for as long as it takes for their digestive symptoms to subside. Once digestive symptoms have abated, she says they can move on to the full GAPS diet and add more foods.

"Your patient needs to have at least six months of normal digestion before you start introducing foods not allowed on the GAPS diet," she says. "Do not rush with this step." Some people may take longer than two years to be able to accommodate non-GAPS foods. The first foods to introduce once you're ready to come off the diet include new potatoes and fermented gluten-free grains.

Dr. Campbell-McBride urges those considering the GAPS diet to follow it strictly according to the blueprint in her book. That makes it difficult to modify. Vegetarians may find the diet tricky to follow since the diet relies on animal-based protein.

However, the diet is naturally gluten-free, corn-free, and peanut-free, and easily can be made dairy-free if you have an allergy or an intolerance to dairy foods. Those with a tree nut allergy will need to avoid certain recipes, but shouldn't have much trouble finding foods they can eat on the diet.

Following the GAPS diet means you'll cook almost all your own food from scratch. In many cases, you'll use homemade meat or fish stock for soups, broths, and other recipes. Dr. Campbell-McBride believes that homemade stock has a "soothing effect" on areas of inflammation within the intestinal tract. Commercial stock products don't have this same effect, according to Dr. Camobell-McBride.

How to follow the GAPS diet

To follow the GAPS diet, eliminate grains, sugar, soy, pasteurized dairy, starchy vegetables, and processed foods from the diet.

The diet is restrictive and may take up to 2 years to complete.

There are three stages to the GAPS diet:

1. The introduction diet

PinterestA person can add avocado at stage 3 of the introduction diet.

Dr. Campbell-McBride recommends that many people follow the introduction diet before starting the full GAPS diet.

While highly restrictive, this phase aims to heal the gut and reduce digestive symptoms quickly. It can last anywhere from a few weeks to 1 year.

The introduction diet has six progressive stages. Each stage introduces new foods but foods within each stage are individualized to each person based on tolerance.

People should not progress to the next stage if they experience digestive symptoms, which may include:

- diarrhea

- bloating

- gas

- constipation

- abdominal pain

Stage 1

In stage 1, the diet consists of:

- homemade meat stock

- boiled meat or fish

- well-cooked vegetables

- probiotics, such as fermented vegetable juices, yogurt or kefir, and homemade fermented whey

- ginger or chamomile tea with raw honey

- purified water

Stage 2

In stage 2, add the following foods:

- raw, organic egg yolks

- casseroles made with meats and vegetables

- fermented fish

- homemade ghee

Stage 3

In stage 3, add the following foods:

- avocado

- sauerkraut and fermented vegetables

- GAPS pancakes

- scrambled eggs made with ghee, goose fat, or duck fat

- probiotic supplements

Stage 4

In stage 4, add the following foods:

- roasted or grilled meats

- cold-pressed olive oil

- freshly pressed carrot juice

- GAPS milkshake

- GAPS bread

Stage 5

In stage 5, add the following foods:

• cooked apple purée

• raw vegetables, such as lettuce and peeled cucumber

• pressed fruit juice

Stage 6

In stage 6, add the following foods:

• raw, peeled apple

• raw fruit

• increase honey

• baked goods sweetened with dried fruit

After completing the introduction diet, many people move onto the full GAPS diet.

2. The full GAPS diet

During the GAPS diet, avoid all grains, sugars, starchy vegetables, refined carbohydrates, and processed foods. This stage lasts 18–24 months but is individualized and may require less time for some.

Acceptable GAPS foods include:

- eggs

- meat, fish, and shellfish (fresh or frozen only)

- fresh vegetables and fruit

- garlic

- natural fats, such as olive oil, coconut oil, and ghee

- a moderate amount of nuts

- GAPS baked goods made using nut flour

The GAPS diet also recommends that people:

- use organic food as often as possible

- avoid all processed and packaged foods

- eat fermented food with every meal

- drink bone broth with every meal

- avoid eating fruit with meals

- combine all protein food with vegetables, which the theory says will keep body acidity levels normal

3. The reintroduction phase

After at least 6 months of normal digestion, people can choose to move on to the reintroduction phase.

The final stage of the GAPS diet involves gradually reintroducing food items over the course of several months.

The diet recommends starting with potatoes and fermented grains. Start with small portions and gradually increase the amount of food, as long as no digestive issues arise. Continue this process with starchy vegetables, grains, and beans.

After completing the GAPS diet, many people continue to avoid refined, highly processed foods.

How to Know if You Need the GAPS Diet

It's not only those with poor digestion who should consider the GAPS Diet. If you'd like to see one or more of these health improvements, then this diet just might be for you:

- Reduced food allergies or sensitivities

- Cured candida yeast

- Improved neurological/cognitive functions

- Reversed Type II Diabetes

- Lose resistant extra weight

- Improved detoxification process

- Improved symptoms of autism

- Reduced anxiety and depression

- Cleared up skin conditions such as eczema, acne, dermatitis or psoriasis

- Reduced chronic constipation or diarrhea

- Improved asthma or chronic sinus infections

- Cured acid reflux

- Reduced seasonal allergy symptoms

Can the GAPS diet help you lose weight?

The GAPS plan is not a weight-loss diet, and it's most definitely not a quick fix approach. It's meant to be followed carefully and long-term. While encouraged by some practitioners, it requires a huge commitment and cannot offer any data or statistics related to its promises.

If you're still thinking of trying GAPS, talk to your physician first, especially if you've been diagnosed with any of the conditions the diet can supposedly cure. If your MD supports your decision to move forward, work with a registered dietitian, who can guide you in properly following the plan, assess your intake to be sure you're meeting your nutrient needs, and monitor your progress.

The Nuts and Bolts of the GAPS Diet

The GAP Diet:

- Provides nutrient-dense foods that restore nutrient deficiencies

- Removes complex carbohydrates that continually "feed" pathogenic bacteria in the body

- Focuses on fermented foods and probiotic supplements to restore a healthy gut flora balance

Scientific studies prove that 80% of our immune system is in our gut and that every kind of autoimmune disease has a connection with leaky gut—a permeable intestinal lining. A leaky gut allows bacterial toxins and undigested food elements to seep into the bloodstream instead of being detoxified or digested. This creates an inflammatory response in the body, causing antibodies to be released where they surround your healthy tissue. The end result is that your entire body becomes inflamed.

The GAPS Diet allows your gut to repair itself by removing the foods that perpetuate leaky gut and rebuild body tissue through dense nutrition. Once the gut is "resealed," the removed foods can slowly be reintroduced back into your diet.

What To Eat?

The GAPS diet begins with an introductory phase (with very limited food selection) followed by a full diet phase, which allows a wider variety of foods. Dr. Campbell-McBride urges everyone to try the introductory phase before moving on to the entire diet. However, she states that those whose conditions are particularly severe may need to stay in the introductory phase for longer.

The introductory phase allows only homemade meat, chicken, or fish stock; a homemade soup made with stock plus non-starchy vegetables; homemade fermented foods such as sauerkraut or vegetables; homemade fermented dairy products; organic egg yolks; and avocado.

Gradually, as digestive symptoms subside, you can add pancakes made from nut butter and vegetables; homemade ghee; fried eggs; roasted and grilled meats; olive oil; bread made with almond flour; cooked apple; raw vegetables; homemade juice; and raw apples.

Once the person can eat all of those items without digestive symptoms, then they're ready for the full GAPS protocol. It takes at least one-and-a-half to two years on the GAPS diet protocol before those following the plan can begin to eat non-compliant foods again.

Food to Eat

- Meat, poultry, fish, and eggs

- Non-starchy vegetables

- Most fruit

- Fermented dairy (yogurt, kefir, and ghee)

- Fermented fish (using GAPS recipe)

- Fermented vegetables

- Homemade vegetable and fruit juice

- Nuts, nut butters, and nut flour

- Butter

- Olive oil

- Coconut oil

- Honey

Food to avoid

- All grains (e.g., wheat, rice, barley, oats, and corn) and grain products (e.g., bread, breakfast cereal, and pasta)

- Starchy vegetables (including potatoes, parsnips, yams, and sweet potatoes)

- Quinoa, buckwheat, sorghum, millet, and other "gluten-free" grains

- Sugar and anything that contains it

- Maple syrup, molasses, corn syrup, and any other syrup

• Aspartame in any form and any food that contains it

• Candy, cookies, cakes, and ice cream

• Milk (unless it's fermented)

• All processed foods

• All alcoholic beverages

Here's a rundown of the foods that are allowed (and aren't allowed) on the GAPS diet protocol.

Food to Eat

Meats, Poultry, and Fish

The GAPS diet protocol allows all types of animal protein. However, you'll need to cook them and serve them only with allowed sauces and spices, which means you'll be making them at home for the most part.

Non-Starchy Vegetables

Some vegetables are allowed, some are not. Non-starchy vegetables are encouraged on the GAPS diet—in fact, you're urged to ferment them using recipes and cultures that are "GAPS-approved." Non-starchy vegetables include carrots, onions, asparagus, broccoli, cabbage, Brussels sprouts, cauliflower, kale, Swiss chard, lettuce, and beets.

Fruit

Virtually all fruits are allowed. Bananas are the only type of fruit that comes with a modification on the diet: They must be very ripe. If they have brown spots on them, they're ready.

Fermented Foods

Foods that have been fermented also are recommended as a source of beneficial bacteria. Dr. Campbell-McBride's book includes recipes for sauerkraut, fermented vegetables, and fermented probiotic beverages.

Food to avoid

Grains

These include multiple foods that are staples in most people's diets, including bread, cereal, crackers, pasta, cakes, cookies, and all other conventional baked goods. Dr. Campbell-McBride believes that these foods irritate the gut lining and ultimately damage it, which affects how nutrients are absorbed.

Dairy Products

Only fermented dairy products are allowed in most cases. Milk—particularly cow's milk—can irritate and damage the intestinal lining in much the same way as grains do, according to Dr. Campbell-McBride's theory. Fermented versions of dairy-based foods do not have this effect. As a result, the dairy-based foods allowed on the GAPS diet are almost all homemade fermented foods: yogurt, kefir, ghee, and whey. The exception is butter, which is allowed.

Starchy Vegetables

Vegetables that are not allowed on the diet include potatoes, sweet potatoes, parsnips, and yams. Beans and legumes are also not allowed on the GAPS diet.

Sugar and Added Sugars

On the GAPs diet, sugar is considered harmful to the gut lining. The ban on sugar and artificial sweeteners (and on ingredients such as maple syrup, molasses, and aspartame) means you'll need to steer clear of foods with added sugars, too.

Processed Foods and Alcohol

All processed foods (with the exception of the very few that are specifically labeled "GAPS-compliant") contain ingredients that are off-limits on the diet. In addition, alcoholic beverages are not allowed.

GAPS supplements

The diet's founder states that the most important aspect of the GAPS protocol is the diet.

However, the GAPS protocol also recommends various supplements. These include:

- probiotics

- essential fatty acids

- digestive enzymes

- cod liver oil

Probiotics

Probiotic supplements are added to the diet to help restore the balance of beneficial bacteria in your gut.

It's recommended that you choose a probiotic containing strains from a range of bacteria, including Lactobacilli, Bifidobacteria, and Bacillus subtilis varieties.

You're advised to look for a product that contains at least 8 billion bacterial cells per gram and to introduce the probiotic slowly into your diet.

Essential fatty acids and cod liver oil

People on the GAPS diet are advised to take daily supplements of both fish oil and cod liver oil to ensure they're getting enough.

The diet also suggests you take small amounts of a cold-pressed nut and seed oil blend that has a 2:1 ratio of omega-3 to omega-6 fatty acids.

Digestive enzymes

The diet's founder claims that people with GAPS conditions also have low stomach acid production. To remedy this, she suggests followers of the diet take a supplement of betaine HCl with added pepsin before each meal.

This supplement is a manufactured form of hydrochloric acid, one of the main acids produced in your stomach. Pepsin is an enzyme also produced in the stomach, which works to break down and digest proteins.

Some people may want to take additional digestive enzymes to support digestion.

Benefits

Healthy Home-Cooked Meals

The GAPS diet encourages home-cooked meals made from fresh vegetables, fruits, meats, poultry, and fish. No restaurant-made food is allowed on the diet. This means the GAPS diet will be a healthier diet than the typical American diet.

May Help Treat Symptoms

Some proponents of the diet, including its creator, claim that it can help improve symptoms of autism, ADHD, and other mental health conditions in children and adults who follow it. Dr. Campbell-McBride maintains a list of physicians whom she has trained on the diet, though there is limited evidence to prove its efficacy.

Drawbacks

Limited Evidence

Like other diet treatments for autism, the GAPS diet does not have any rigorous medical studies to back it up. Unfortunately, there's little scientific evidence to indicate that any of Dr. Campbell-McBride's recommendations—ranging from homemade broth to fermented foods—can help improve symptoms of autism or other mental health conditions.

Restrictive and Time-Consuming

Because of its restrictive nature, the GAPS diet is extremely difficult to follow. You'll need to cook all your own food from scratch—no store-bought convenience foods, such as broth or most sauces, are allowed. This means you will spend a lot of time in the kitchen, which your lifestyle may or may not allow.

The GAPS diet food list

The GAPS diet eliminates all grains and legumes and emphasizes animal protein, homemade bone broth, non-starchy vegetables, and fermented foods. The following sample shopping list provides suggestions for getting started with this eating plan. Note that this list is not all-inclusive and there may be other foods that work better for you.

- Leafy greens (bok choy, collard greens, kale, green leaf lettuce, spinach)

- Non-starchy vegetables (asparagus, Brussels sprouts, broccoli, cabbage, cauliflower, avocados, cucumbers, green beans, okra, zucchini)

- Fruits (berries, oranges, pineapple, banana, grapefruit, raisins)

- Meat and poultry (lean cuts of beef, ground beef, whole chicken, chicken breast, turkey breast)

- Fish (salmon, halibut, cod, tuna, mackerel, sea bass)

- Fermented dairy products (yogurt, kefir, ghee)

- Fermented vegetables (pickled sauerkraut, kimchi)

- Nuts (almonds, cashews, hazelnuts, pistachios, walnuts)

- Nut butters (almond, cashew, hazlenut)

- Nut flours (almond flour/meal, hazelnut flour/meal)

- Olive oil, coconut oil

- Butter

- Honey

- Fresh herbs (thyme, rosemary)

- Eggs

Sample Meal Plan

A key tenet of the GAPS diet is making all or most of your own meals from scratch, including nourishing bone broths and fruit juices. The following three-day meal plan provides suggestions for what to eat on the GAPS protocol. Note that this plan is not all-inclusive, and if you choose to follow this diet there may be other foods that are more appropriate for your tastes and preferences.

Day 1

- Breakfast: 1 cup yogurt topped with 1 cup mixed berries; 8 ounces fresh-squeezed orange juice

- Lunch: 1 cup Chicken, Vegetable, and Ginger Soup (substitute homemade broth for the stock)

- Dinner: 1 1/4 cup Chinese-Style Beef and Broccoli; 1/2 cup kimchi

Day 2

- Breakfast: 2 eggs, scrambled or over-easy; 2 strips turkey bacon; 1/2 cup sauerkraut

- Lunch: 1 1/4 cups Beef and Mushroom Soup (omit brown rice; substitute homemade broth for the stock); 1 1/2 cups Kale and Cranberry Green Salad (omit feta)

• Dinner: 4 ounces Oven-Baked Salmon With Herbs; 1 serving Roasted Asparagus

Day 3

• Breakfast: 2 Almond Meal Pancakes topped with half a sliced banana and a tablespoon of almond butter

• Lunch: 1 Tuna Salad Collard Green Wrap (omit mayo); 1 serving (28 g) walnuts

• Dinner: 1 serving Roasted Chicken With Turmeric and Fennel; 1 cup cauliflower "rice"

GAPS DIET RECIPES

Trying gaps-friendly recipes is a great way to explore new flavors and find new favorite dishes while looking after your health. In this part are nourishing gaps diet recipes for you to enjoy.

Superfood Meatballs

Preparation time

45 minutes

Ingredients

- 1- 1.5 lb grassfed ground beef

- 2-4 oz grassfed beef liver

- 1 medium onion

- 1 tsp real salt

- Stock pot full of meat stock

Instructions

1. Rinse the liver and place it in a bowl of cool water, along with a tsp of fresh lemon juice or apple cider vinegar. This helps to lessen the bitter taste.

2. Let sit for half an hour.

3. Chop the onion intro fairly small pieces.

4. Mix the ground beef, salt and onion together in a large bowl.

5. Bring the stock to a boil.

6. Remove liver from lemon juice soak and rinse.

7. Place liver in high powered blender or food processor and blend until it is pureed.

8. Add the liver to the ground beef mixture and mix well.

9. Turn the meat stock down to a simmer.

10. Begin forming balls with the meat about 1-2 Tbsp in size, then gently drop in the simmering meat stock.

11. Continuing forming and dropping meatballs into the stock until you've used all of the meat.

12. Cook for approximately 20-30 minutes; adding veggies, if desired, to serve as a soup or stew, or ladle out meatballs to serve alongside vegetables.

Three Cup Chicken

Preparation time

30 minutes

Ingredients

• 3 Tbsp toasted sesame oil

• One (3-inch) piece fresh ginger, peeled and sliced into matchsticks

• 15-20 medium garlic cloves, peeled and smashed (with the side of a knife)

• 1 tsp freshly ground black pepper

• 1 pinch ground cloves

- 2 pounds skin-on, bone-in chicken drumsticks and/or thighs; chopped into 1-2 inch pieces if desired

- 1/2 cup rice wine

- 3 tbsp coconut aminos

- 1 tbsp fish sauce

- 1 tbsp honey

- 2 cups fresh Thai basil leaves

- Steamed white rice or cauliflower rice, for serving

Instructions

1. Heat a large skillet or wok over high heat.

2. Add sesame oil.

3. Add the ginger, garlic, pepper, and cloves and saute until fragrant, about 2 minutes.

4. Add the chicken, and cook, turning occasionally, until it is browned and crisping at the edges, approximately 5 to 7 minutes.

5. Add honey, stir to combine, and then add the rice wine, coconut aminos, and fish sauce. Bring just to a boil.

6. Lower the heat and simmer until the sauce has reduced and started to thicken, approximately 15 minutes.

7. Turn off the heat, add the basil and stir to combine.

8. Serve with white or cauli rice.

Pesto Sausage Cakes

Prepartion time

15 minutes

Ingredients

- 1 lb. ground pork, chicken or turkey

- 1/2 cup pesto (My pesto is nut and dairy free. It is just peas, evoo, salt and garlic blended together. Use whatever kind you like.)

- 1 egg

- 1 egg yolk

- 1/4 cup bread crumbs or coconut flour (optional, but it helps bind things together)

- salt, garlic powder, cumin to taste

- bread crumbs or coconut flour to coat (optional)

- fat for cooking (palm shortening, coconut oil, lard, butter)

Instructions

1. Mix meat, pesto, eggs, bread crumbs and seasoning.

2. Form into 8-10 patties.

3. Coat patties in bread crumbs or coconut flour.

4. Heat fat in skillet over medium heat.

5. Cook patties in fat until cooked through, about 8 minutes per side.

6. Serve with extra pesto or pesto mayo (mix equal parts pesto and mayo).

SPAGHETTI WITH NO-TOMATO SAUCE

Preparation time

1 hour 10 minutes

Ingredients

SPAGHETTI

- 1 pound ground beef

- 1 teaspoon dried oregano

- 1 teaspoon dried parsley

- 1 teaspoon dried basil

- 1/2 teaspoon ground ginger

- 1/2 teaspoon sea salt

- 4 cups no-tomato sauce (below)

- 4 cups spinach (chopped)

- 1 whole spaghetti squash (cooked)

NO-TOMATO SAUCE

- 16 medium carrot (chopped)

- 8 cloves garlic (chopped)

- 4 small onion (chopped)

- 2 medium beet (chopped)

- 8 whole bay leaf

- 2 cups chicken broth

- 2 tablespoons dried basil

- 2 tablespoons dried thyme

- 1 tablespoon dried rosemary

- 1 tablespoon dried parsley

- 1 tablespoons dried oregano

- 1 tablespoon sea salt (or to taste)

Instructions

SPAGHETTI

1. Brown the meat with oregano, parsley, basil, ginger, and salt in a large skillet over medium heat.

2. Add the no-tomato sauce and bring to a boil.

3. Reduce the heat and simmer for 1 hour, stirring occasionally.

4. Stir in the spinach and cook until its reduced, then serve over the spaghetti squash.

NO-TOMATO SAUCE

1. Combine all ingredients in a slow cooker and cook on low for 7 hours.

2. Remove the bay leaves.

3. Puree in a blender until smooth, then season to taste.

Slow Cooker Honey Garlic Chicken

Preparation time

5 hours

Ingredients:

- 2 Chicken Breasts

- 1 TBS of Olive Oil

- 1 TBS Apple Cider Vinegar

- 1 TBS of Honey

- 3 cloves of garlic (minced or chopped)

- salt to taste

Instructions

1. Place chicken breasts in the crock-pot, in a small bowl add the remaining ingredients and stir until combined.

2. Pour the combined ingredients over the chicken.

3. Cook in slow cooker on high for 3-5 hours.

ROAST BEEF TENDERLOIN

Preparation time

8 hours

Ingredients

- 1 4-5 pound beef tenderloin, trimmed (if you'd like a small roast and one that's pastured, I highly recommend this one)

- 1 cup fermented tamari or coconut aminos

- 1/4 cup red wine vinegar

- 2 tablespoons ground garlic

- ?1 tablespoon freshly ground black pepper

- 2 tablespoons ghee , tallow ,or lard

Instructions

1. Place the tenderloin in a shallow baking dish.

2. Stir together tamari and vinegar and pour over the roast.

3. Season the meat with all the garlic and black pepper.

4. Marinate for 4 hours, rotating after 2 hours.

5. Let the roast sit at room temperature for 1 hour before cooking.

6. Preheat the oven to 425ºF and adjust the rack to the middle position.

7. Place a large skillet over medium-high heat for 2 minutes.

8. Add the ghee and swirl the pan to coat.

9. Place the roast on the skillet and cook for 3-4 minutes until bottom is turning golden brown.

10. Using a pair of tongs, turn the meat and cook for another 3-4 minutes until golden brown.

11. Repeat this until all 4 sides are seared.

12. Transfer the roast to a large baking sheet, insert the thermometer in the thickest part of the roast and place in the oven.

13. Roast for about 25-35 minutes, until thermometer reads 125ºF for medium-rare.

14. Remove from the oven and let the meat rest for 10 minutes before serving.

LEMON-THYME ROASTED CHICKEN THIGHS

Prepartion time

30 minutes

Ingredients

- Zest from 1 lemon

- 1 tablespoon fresh lemon juice

- 2 cloves garlic, minced

- 1 tablespoon chopped cilantro

- 1 tablespoon chopped thyme

- 1/2 teaspoon Celtic Sea salt

- 4 bone-in, skin-on organic chicken thighs

- 2 tablespoons ghee , melted (or duck fat for dairy-free)

Instructions

1. Preheat the oven to 425ºF and adjust the rack to the middle position.

2. Place a wire cooling rack over a baking sheet.

3. Combine the lemon zest, juice, garlic, cilantro, thyme, and sea salt in a small bowl and stir to combine.

4. Loosen the skin on the chicken things and insert about 1 tablespoon of lemon mixture under skin of each.

5. Brush each chicken thigh (bottom and top of thigh) with ghee and place on the wire rack.

6. Roast the chicken until the skin is golden brown and crisp and a thermometer inserted into

the thickest part of the chicken, but not touching

the bone registers 165ºF, about 20-25 minutes.

7. Remove the chicken from the oven and let it

rest for 5 minutes.

8. Serve.

Slow-Cooked Greens with Garlic

Prepartion time

1 hour 10 minutes

Ingredients:

• 2 pounds Tuscan kale (you can also use Swiss

chard), ribs and stems removed and torn into

large bite-size pieces, roughly 2-inches in diameter each

- 4 tablespoons unsalted butter

- 4 cloves garlic, minced

- 1/4 teaspoon red chili flakes

- 1/2 teaspoon Celtic sea salt

- 1 tablespoon fresh lemon juice

Instructions

1. Bring a large pot of water to boil.

2. Place the kale in the water and boil for 8 minutes.

3. Drain and then squeeze out the excess water.

4. Melt the butter in a large skillet over medium heat.

5. Add the garlic and red chili flakes and cook until fragrant, about 45 seconds.

6. Add the cooked kale, reduce heat to medium-low and cook, stirring occasionally, for 20-25 minutes until deep green and tender.

7. Remove from the heat and season with salt and stir in lemon juice.

8. Serve.

ROASTED SALMON WITH CHIMMICHURRI (GRAIN-FREE, PALEO)

Prepartion time

21 minutes

Ingredients

For the salmon:

- 4 skin-on wild salmon fillets

- Celtic Sea salt

For the Chimichurri:

- 1 cup fresh flat-leaf parsley leaves

- 1 cup fresh cilantro

- 3 cloves garlic

- 1/2 cup extra virgin olive oil

- 1/4 cup red wine vinegar

- 1 teaspoon Celtic Sea salt

Instructions

1. Preheat the oven to 400ºF and adjust the rack to the middle position.

2. Place the salmon on a baking dish lined with parchment paper.

3. Sprinkle with Celtic Sea salt.

4. Place the salmon in the oven and roast for 11 minutes.

5. Meanwhile, place the parsley, cilantro, garlic, and sea salt in a food processor and pulse until coarsely chopped, about 5 one-second pulses.

6. Add the olive oil and vinegar and pulse, until combined, about 5 one-second pulses.

7. Transfer to bowl; set aside.

8. Spoon the chimichurri over top of each salmon fillet and serve.

ROASTED BUTTERNUT SQUASH WITH GOAT CHEESE AND PECANS

Prepartion time

55 minutes

Ingredients

- 1 2-3 pound butternut squash, skin and seeds removed and cut into 1/2" thick slices

- 3 tablespoons ghee , melted

- 1/2 teaspoon Celtic sea salt

- 1/8 teaspoon cayenne

- 1/4 cup goat cheese, crumbled

- 1/2 cup pecans, toasted and chopped

- 1 teaspoon fresh thyme leaves

Instructions

1. Preheat the oven to 425ºF and adjust the rack to the lowest position.

2.   Place the squash in a large bowl and toss with the ghee, sea salt and cayenne.

3.   Spread the squash in an even layer on a baking sheet lined with parchment paper.

4. Roast for 25-30 minutes until well browned.

5. Remove the squash from the oven and, using a pair of tongs, flip each piece of squash.

6.   Then, continue to roast in the oven until the face-down side of the squash is browned, about 10 more minutes.

7. Transfer the squash to a platter and top with the goat cheese, pecans and fresh thyme.

8. Serve warm.

BUTTERNUT SQUASH, CARROT AND COCONUT SOUP (GRAIN-FREE)

Prepartion time

1 hour 40 minutes

Ingredients

For the Squash:

- 2 pounds butternut squash, peeled, seeded and cut into 2-inch chunks

- 1 tablespoon ghee , melted (you can substitute palm shortening for a dairy-free option)

For the Soup:

- 2 tablespoons unsalted butter (or coconut oil)

- 3 carrots, cut into 1/4" thick coins

- 1 leek, white and light parts only, chopped

- 1/2 teaspoon dried thyme

- 1 1/2 teaspoons Celtic sea salt

- 3 cups chicken broth (you can use bone broth or meat stock)

- 1 cup coconut milk

Instructions

1. Preheat the oven to 400ºF and adjust the rack to the middle position.

2. Place the squash on a baking sheet lined with unbleached parchment paper .

3. Pour the ghee overtop and gently toss to coat the squash.

4. Roast for 30 minutes, or until soft when pierced with a knife.

5. Meanwhile, melt the butter in a large pot over low heat.

6. Add the carrots and leeks and stir to combine.

7. Put the lid on the pot and let the vegetables sweat for 30 minutes.

8. After 30 minutes, remove the lid and stir in the thyme and sea salt.

9. Add the chicken broth and roasted squash to the carrot mixture and bring to a simmer.

10. Then, using an immersion blender, blend the soup until smooth.

11. Or, you can also process the soup in a blender until smooth.

12. Stir in the coconut milk.

13. Season to taste with sea salt.

14. Serve.

Note:

- I like butternut squash soup on the creamier side, but if you like it a bit thinner, than just add 1/2 cup or so of water.

LEMON CREAM POTS

Prepartion time

4 hours 20 minutes

Ingredients

• 2 cups raw cream or organic heavy cream (this recipe does not work with dairy-free milk alternatives)

• 3 tablespoons raw honey

• 1 tablespoon lemon zest

• 1/4 cup fresh lemon juice

• 1/4 cup whipped cream (optional)

Instructions

1. Place the cream and honey in a saucepan over medium heat and stir until the honey is dissolved.

2. Bring the mixture to a boil and cook for 3 minutes.

3. Remove from the heat and stir in the lemon rind and juice.

4. Cool for 5 minutes then pour into four small serving bowls.

5. Place in the refrigerator and chill for 4 hours until set.

6. Serve with a dollop of whipped cream.

TORTILLA SOUP RECIPE

Prepartion time

45 minutes

Ingredients

For the soup:

• 5 cloves garlic, crushed with skins on

• 6 springs fresh oregano

• 6 sprigs of cilantro, plus 1/2 cup roughly chopped

• 8 cups chicken stock

• 2 pounds bone-in chicken breasts or 1 small 3-4 pound chicken

For the Toppings:

- 3 cups Siete tortilla chips

- 1 avocado, cubed

- 2 tomatoes, cut into bite-size chunks

- 1 lime, cut into quarters

- 1/2 cup sour cream (omit for Paleo and Gaps)

- 1/2 cup shredded cheddar cheese (omit for Paleo)

Instructions

1. Place the garlic cloves in a large dutch oven over medium-high heat.

2. Cook, stirring frequently until garlic begins to darken, about 2-2 1/2 minutes.

3. Remove the pot from the heat and let it cool for about 30 seconds and then add the chicken stock, oregano, cilantro, and chicken to the garlic.

4. Place pot back on heat and bring to a boil and then reduce to a simmer.

5. Simmer for about 30 minutes.

6. When chicken is cooked through, remove the chicken from the broth mixture and set aside.

7. With slotted spoon, strain out the rest of the garlic and herbs.

8. Shred the chicken with a fork and then add back to the soup.

9. Add salt and pepper if needed.

10. To serve, crumble a handful of tortilla chips into individual bowls and then ladle the broth over.

11. Serve with cilantro, avocado, tomatoes, lime, cheese, and sour cream.

MEAT STOCK – WHAT TO DRINK IF YOU CAN'T TOLERATE BONE BROTH

Prepartion time

4 hours 5 minutes

Ingredients

- 1 whole 3-4 pound raw chicken

- 1 yellow onion, cut in half

- 1 head garlic, cut in half

- 1 carrot

- 1 piece of celery

- 1 tablespoon apple cider vinegar

Instructions

1. Place all of the ingredients in a large pot and cover with water. Heat over low heat until it reaches a simmer. Continue to simmer on low for 3-4 hours. Strain. Pour the stock into glass jars and store in the refrigerator.

Dairy free green Goddess dressing

Prepartion time

8 hours 15 minutes

Ingredients

For the Cashews:

- 3/4 cups cashews

For the Dressing:

- 3/4 cups water

- 1 cup chopped green onion, white and green parts

- 1 cup chopped fresh basil leaves

- 1/4 cup freshly squeezed lemon juice

- 2 cloves garlic, chopped

- 2 anchovy fillets or 2 teaspoons anchovy paste

- 1 teaspoon Celtic sea salt

- 1 teaspoon freshly ground black pepper

Instructions

1. The night before, place the cashews in a bowl and cover with water and a pinch of sea salt. Let sit at room temperature overnight. The next day, or at least 8 hours later, drain the cashews and place in a blender. Add the 3/4 cup of water and blend until smooth. Add the remaining ingredients and blend until smooth. Store in a mason jar in the refrigerator.

SALMON AND BABY GREENS SALAD WITH CREAMY GARLIC DRESSING

Preparation time

Ingredients

For the onions:

- 1 red onion, sliced thin

- 1/2 cup white wine vinegar

- 1/2 cup apple cider vinegar

- 1/2 teaspoon raw honey

- 1/4 teaspoon Celtic sea salt

For the salmon:

1. 12 ounces wild salmon fillet, cut into 4 pieces

2. Celtic sea salt

3. Freshly ground black pepper

For the salad:

• 8 ounces baby lettuces

• 1/2 English cucumber, sliced

• 1/4 cup capers

• 1/4 cup sprouted pumpkin seeds

• 1/2 pint cherry tomatoes, each cut in half

For the dressing:

- 1/3-3/4 cup garlic-yogurt dressing (depending on how saturated you like your salad to be)

Instructions

1. Place the red onion, vinegars, honey and sea salt in a mason jar. Screw the lid on and shake until combined. Unscrew the lid and, using a spoon, press down the onions so they are all submerged in the liquid. Set aside for at least 30 minutes. (Can be made 1-6 days ahead of time and stored in the refrigerator.)

2. Preheat the oven to 450ºF and adjust the rack to the middle position. Season the salmon with sea salt and pepper. Place the salmon, skin down, on a baking sheet lined with unbleached

parchment paper. Roast, 12 minutes, until salmon is cooked through.

3. To assemble the salad, place the lettuces, cucumber, capers, pumpkin seeds, cherry tomatoes and 1/2 cup of pickled onions in a large salad bowl. Pour the dressing over top and toss. Using salad tongs, divide the salad onto four plates. Top with salmon and serve.

BRAISED CHICKEN THIGHS WITH SQUASH AND KALE (GRAIN-FREE)

Prepartion time

Ingredients

- 4 pounds skin-on, bone-in chicken thighs (about 12), patted dry

- Celtic sea salt

- Freshly ground pepper

- 2 tablespoons ghee

- 1 bunch scallions, sliced into 1-inch pieces

- 1 dried chiles de árbol

- 2 tablespoons chopped ginger

- 3 cups chicken broth, divided

- 1/2 cup fermented gluten-free tamari or coconut aminos

- 2 tablespoons coconut sugar (or raw honey for GAPS)

- 2 tablespoons sesame oil

- 1 butternut squash, cut into bite-size pieces

- 1 bunch kale, chopped and steamed (this is why I prefer to cook the greens first, but if you'd like to add them raw, that will work as well)

- 1 tablespoon coconut vinegar

- 2 teaspoons toasted sesame seeds

Instructions

1. Lightly season the chicken thighs with sea salt and pepper. Heat the ghee in a large Dutch oven or other heavy pot over medium-high. Working in 2 batches, cook chicken, skin side down, until skin is browned and crisp, about 8–10 minutes. Transfer the chicken to a plate, placing skin side up (the chicken will not be cooked through at this point).

2. Keep the heat at medium-high (keep any leftover ghee, chicken fat, etc. in the pot) and place the scallions, chiles, and ginger in the pot to cook, stirring frequently until onions are just turning golden brown on the edges, about 3 minutes.

3. Add 1 cup of chicken broth , bring to a simmer, and cook until reduced to about 3

tablespoons. This will take about 5 minutes. Add the tamari, coconut sugar, sesame oil, and remaining broth and bring to a simmer, stirring to dissolve sugar. Place the butternut squash and kale in the pot. Place the chicken, skin-side up on top of the squash and kale, and, using a pair of tongs, nestle each piece of chicken down into the liquid mixture so the bottom of each piece of chicken is in the liquid. Partially cover the pot, reduce the heat to medium-low, and simmer until the chicken and squash are cooked through, about 20 minutes.

4. Remove the chicken, increase the heat to medium, and continue to cook until liquid is reduced by about two-thirds and has the consistency of thin gravy, about 10–15 minutes.

5. Remove the pot from heat and drizzle the vinegar over the squash and kale mixture. Add the chicken back to pot, turning to coat in sauce, and sprinkle sesame seeds over top.

6. This recipe can be made 2 days ahead. Let cool; cover and chill and then reheat covered over low heat.

TORTILLA SOUP RECIPE

Preparation time

45 minutes

Ingredients

For the soup:

- 5 cloves garlic, crushed with skins on

- 6 springs fresh oregano

- 6 sprigs of cilantro, plus 1/2 cup roughly chopped

- 8 cups chicken stock

- 2 pounds bone-in chicken breasts or 1 small 3-4 pound chicken

For the Toppings:

- 3 cups Siete tortilla chips

- 1 avocado, cubed

- 2 tomatoes, cut into bite-size chunks

- 1 lime, cut into quarters

- 1/2 cup sour cream (omit for Paleo and Gaps)

- 1/2 cup shredded cheddar cheese (omit for Paleo)

Instructions

1. Place the garlic cloves in a large dutch oven over medium-high heat.

2. Cook, stirring frequently until garlic begins to darken, about 2-2 1/2 minutes.

3. Remove the pot from the heat and let it cool for about 30 seconds and then add the chicken stock, oregano, cilantro, and chicken to the garlic.

4. Place pot back on heat and bring to a boil and then reduce to a simmer.

5. Simmer for about 30 minutes.

6. When chicken is cooked through, remove the chicken from the broth mixture and set aside.

7. With slotted spoon, strain out the rest of the garlic and herbs.

8. Shred the chicken with a fork and then add back to the soup.

9. Add salt and pepper if needed.

10. To serve, crumble a handful of tortilla chips into individual bowls and then ladle the broth over.

11. Serve with cilantro, avocado, tomatoes, lime, cheese, and sour cream.

EASY SLOW COOKER PEPPER STEAK

(GRAIN-FREE, PALEO)

Prepartion time

6 hours 10 minutes

Ingredients

• 2 red onions, peeled and cut into wedges

• 1 1/2 pounds chuck roast, cut into bite-size pieces

• 3 red, orange or yellow bell peppers, cut into wedges

• 1 cup chicken broth

• 1/4 cup coconut aminos or gluten-free fermented Tamari

- 1/4 cup tomato paste

- 4 garlic cloves, minced

Instructions

1. Place the onions in the bottom of the slow cooker.

2. Top the onions with the meat and then add the bell peppers.

3. Whisk together the chicken broth, aminos, tomato paste and garlic and pour over the meat mixture.

4. Gently press the vegetables and meat so the meat is submerged in the broth mixture (this helps prevent the meat from drying out).

5. Cook for 6 hours on low.

6. Serve over cauliflower "rice" or soaked rice.

GREEK SALAD WITH BEEF KABOBS

Prepartion time

1 hour 15

Ingredients

For the kabobs:

- 1 pound sirloin, cut into 1 1/2-inch cubes

- 3 tablespoons extra-virgin olive oil

- 1 tablespoon red wine vinegar

- 1/2 teaspoon garlic powder

For the salad:

- 6 ounces baby romaine

- 1/2 red onion, sliced thin

- 1/2 cup Kalamata olives

- 1/2 cup feta cheese, crumbled (omit for dairy
free)

- 1/2 English cucumber, slices

- 1 pint cherry tomatoes, cut in half

For the dressing:

- 1/4 cup extra virgin olive oil

- 2 tablespoons red wine vinegar

- 2 garlic cloves, crushed

- 1/2 teaspoon Celtic sea salt

- Freshly ground black pepper

Instructions

1. Place the sirloin in a flat dish.

2. Whisk together the olive oil, red wine vinegar and garlic in a measuring cup.

3. Pour the marinade over the steak and lift the steak up so the marinade covers the bottom side of the steak as well.

4. Let sit for 1 hour at room temperature, or 2-3 hours in the fridge.

5. Heat the grill to medium (or you can use an indoor grilling pan).

6. Thread the meat onto skewers and grill until medium-rare to medium, depending on your preference.

7. Set aside.

8. Place the romaine, red onion, Kalamata olives and feta cheese, cucumber and tomatoes in a salad bowl.

9. Whisk the olive oil, red wine vinegar, garlic, and sea salt in a measuring cup.

10. Pour the dressing over the salad.

11. Serve the salad with the beef kabobs and season with just a bit of freshly ground black pepper.

GRILLED CHICKEN WITH OLIVE TAPENADE (AND HEALTHY EATING TIPS)

Prepartion time

20 minutes

Ingredients

For the Chicken:

- 4 organic boneless, skinless chicken breasts

- Celtic sea salt and freshly ground black pepper

For the Tapenade:

- 1 cup green olives

- 2 shallots, peeled

- 1 clove garlic

- 1/2 cup flat-leaf parsley

- 1 tablespoon fresh lemon juice

- Zest of 1 lemon

- 1/2 cup extra-virgin olive oil

Instructions

1. Heat the grill to medium and season chicken breasts with sea salt and pepper.

2. Grill until cooked though.

3. Meanwhile, put the green olives, shallots, garlic, parsley, lemon juice and zest in the bowl

of a food processor and pulse until all ingredients are diced.

4. Pour olive mixture into a small bowl and stir in olive oil.

5. Season to taste with sea salt if preferred.

6. Place the grilled chicken on a platter and top with tapenade.

7. Serve.

BUTTER CHICKEN RECIPE

Prepartion time

1 hour 20 minutes

Ingredients

For the marinade:

- 1 cup plain, whole yogurt (or coconut or almond milk yogurt for a dairy-free option)

- 1/4 cup Vindaloo spice blend

- Juice of 1 lemon

- 4 chicken breasts cut into bite-size pieces

For the onions:

- 1 stick unsalted butter (or 4 tablespoons ghee or coconut oil for a dairy-free option)

- 2 yellow onions, thinly sliced

- 1 cup crushed tomatoes

- 1/2 cup chicken stock or broth

- 2 teaspoons Celtic sea salt

- 1/2 cup raw cream or coconut milk

- Cilantro and chopped cashews for serving (optional)

Instructions

1. Stir the yogurt, vindaloo spice blend, and lemon juice together in a medium bowl.

2. Stir in the chicken and make sure the chicken is thoroughly coated with the marinade.

3. Cover and place in the refrigerator to marinate for about 8-10 hours, or you can leave the mixture on the counter for 1 hour to marinate if you're short on time.

4. Melt the butter over low heat in a large sauté pan.

5. Add the onions and cook on low heat for about 35-40 minutes, stirring occasionally until soft and caramelized.

6. Stir in the chicken mixture (yogurt, spices and all) and increase the heat to medium.

7. Stir in the tomatoes, stock and salt.

8. Continue to cook, stirring frequently, until chicken is cooked through, about 15 minutes.

9. Stir in the cream.

10. Serve over riced cauliflower, or soaked brown rice, and top with chopped cilantro and cashews.

SLOW COOKER SPAGHETTI SQUASH WITH MEATBALLS AND MARINARA

Prepartion time

4 hours 15 minutes

Ingredients

For the marinara:

- 2 tablespoons olive oil , plus extra for drizzling

- 1 tablespoon Italian seasoning blend

- 1 (15-ounce) jar crushed tomatoes

- 1 teaspoon Celtic sea salt , plus extra for seasoning

The squash:

- 1 spaghetti squash, cut in half and seeds removed

For the Meatballs:

- 1 pound ground organic turkey

- 1 large egg, beaten (or 2 egg yolks if you need to avoid whites)

- 1/2 teaspoon Celtic sea salt

- 1/4 teaspoon freshly ground black pepper

- Parmesan cheese for garnish (optional)

Instructions

1. Place the olive oil and Italian seasoning in a small sauce pan over medium-low heat. Heat for

about 1 minute, until the herbs are fragrant, then pour into the slow cooker .

2. Add the crushed tomatoes and 1 teaspoon sea salt and stir together.

3. Place the squash halves into the slow cooker, cut side up, on top of the tomato mixture.

4. Season with sea salt and drizzle with a little olive oil.

5. In a medium bowl, combine the turkey, egg, sea salt and black pepper.

6. Using a spoon, scoop bite-size meatballs and place into the tomato mixture.

7. Place the lid on the crock pot and cook on medium heat for 4 hours.

8. Using a fork, remove the spaghetti squash strands from the skins and serve with meatballs and marinara. I like to throw a little parmesan on top!

AVOCADO, MANGO AND PICKLED ONION SALAD WITH JALAPEÑO VINAIGRETTE

Prepartion time

1 hour 10 minutes

Ingredients

For the quick pickled onions:

- 1/2 cup raw apple cider vinegar

- 1 cup filtered water

- 1 teaspoon honey

- 1 teaspoon Celtic sea salt

- 1 red onion, thinly sliced

For the Vinaigrette:

- 1/4 cup fresh lime juice

- 1/4 cup extra-virgin olive oil

- 1/2 jalapeño, seeds removed

- 1 tablespoon chopped red onion

- 1 teaspoon Celtic sea salt

For the Salad:

- 8 cups baby romaine lettuce

- 4 mangoes, cut into bite-size pieces (I prefer Champagne mangos)

- 4 avocados, cut into slices

- 1 recipe picked onions (see recipe above)

Instructions

1. Whisk the apple cider vinegar, water, honey and sea salt together in a measuring cup.

2. Place the onions in a medium bowl and pour the vinegar mixture over the top.

3. Let it sit for 1 hour.

4. Place the lime juice, olive oil, jalapeño, red onion and sea salt in a blender and blend until smooth.

5. Taste and add more salt if you prefer.

6. To Serve: Place the lettuce, mangos, avocados and pickled onions in a large salad bowl (or layer it on a large platter as pictured above).

7. Pour the dressing over the top and toss until coated. Serve immediately.

SHRIMP CEVICHE RECIPE

Prepartion time

45 minutes

Ingredients

• 1 pound raw wild shrimp, peeled and cut into bite-size pieces

• 1/2 cup fresh lime juice

• 1 pint cherry tomatoes, cut in half

• 1/2 cup chopped red onion

• 1/2 cup cucumber, chopped

• 1/2 cup fresh cilantro leaves, chopped

• 1 jalapeno pepper, diveined, seeded and chopped

- 1/2 teaspoon Celtic sea salt

Instructions

1. Place shrimp and lime juice in a shallow dish.

2. Cover, and put in the refrigerator to marinate for 30 minutes.

3. Place tomatoes, red onion, cilantro, jalapeno pepper, sea salt and shrimp and lime mixture in a medium bowl.

4. Stir until incorporated.

5. Season to taste with salt.

6. Serve cold.

CARROTS WITH APRICOTS, HAZELNUTS, AND CREME FRAICHE

Prepartion time

20 minutes

Ingredients

For the Carrots:

- 1 pound carrots, peeled and cut in half-lengthwise

- 2 tablespoons unsalted butter

- 1/2 teaspoon Celtic sea salt

For the Apricots:

- 1/4 cup fresh orange juice

- 1/4 cup chopped dried apricots (I prefer to use unsulphured)

For the Toppings:

- 1/2 cup creme fraiche (can omit if dairy intolerant)

- 1/4 cup chopped hazelnuts (I used soaked and dehydrated nuts)

- 1/4 cup chopped flat-leaf parsley

- 1 tablespoon raw honey

Instructions

1. Melt the butter over medium heat in a large skillet .

2. Place the carrots in one single layer and cook for 4-5 minutes until the edges are turning golden brown.

3. Using a pair of tongs , flip the carrots over and continue cooking until the second side is turning golden brown.

4. If you like the carrots on the crunchier side, then reduce the cooking time by a minute or so per side.

5. Meanwhile, place the orange juice and apricots in a small saucepan and bring to a simmer over low heat.

6. Remove from the heat and drain.

7. To Serve: Spread the creme fraiche on the serving platter.

8. Top with carrots, hazelnuts, parsley, apricots and drizzle with honey.

9. You can also add a bit more of Celtic sea salt if you'd like.

10. Serve immediately.

FERMENTED RADISH SALSA

Prepartion time

48 hours 30 minutes

Ingredients

• 2 bunches radishes, chopped (about 4 cups)

- 2 cups packed cilantro leaves, chopped

- Juice of 2 limes, about 3 tablespoons

- 2 teaspoons Celtic sea salt

Instructions

1. Place all ingredients in a bowl and toss until incorporated.

2. Let sit at room temperature for 20 minutes.

3. Spoon the salsa into a large wide-mouth mason jar .

4. Using a muddler, press the radish mixture so the juices cover the salsa. You might need to press several times to help the juices release from the radishes.

5. Loosely screw the lid on top of the jar.

6. Place the salsa in a dark, cool spot in the pantry.

7. Let sit for 48 hours. You'll notice if you stir the salsa there will be bubbles. That's a good thing! It means the salsa has fermented.

8. Store in the fridge.

CREAM OF VEGETABLE SOUP

Prepartion time

50 minutes

Ingredients

- 4 tablespoons butter (or 3 tablespoons duck fat for a dairy-free option)

- 2 yellow onions, chopped

- 4 carrots, chopped

- 4 large russet potatoes, chopped (or 1 large head cauliflower chopped for a lower carb option)

- 10 cups chicken stock

- 3 sprigs of fresh thyme, tied together with a piece of twine

- 4 zucchini, cut into 1-inch coins

- 2 teaspoons Celtic sea salt

- 1/2 cup raw heavy cream (or coconut milk for a dairy-free option)

- Creme fraiche, sour cream, raw shredded cheddar (optional)

Instructions

1. Melt the butter over low heat in a dutch oven .

2. Add the onions and carrots, put the lid on the pot and let the vegetables sweat for 30 minutes.

3. Add the potatoes and stock and increase heat to medium-high and boil.

4. Reduce the heat to a low boil and cook until potatoes are fork tender.

5. Add the thyme sprigs and zucchini and cook for an additional 8-10 minutes until the zucchini are tender.

6. Remove the thyme bundle from the soup. Using a hand-immersion blender, blend the soup until smooth.

7. Stir in salt and cream. Taste the soup and add more sea salt if needed.

8. Ladle the soup into bowls and serve with a dollop of sour cream or creme fraiche and raw cheddar (if using).

CREAMED KALE WITH SHALLOTS

Prepartion time

30 minutes

Ingredients

- 1 1/2 pounds kale, fibrous stems removed, chopped
- 3 tablespoons unsalted butter (or duck fat or pork lard for a dairy-free option - see above)
- 2 large shallots, sliced (about 1/2 cup)
- 1 clove garlic, finely chopped
- 1 tablespoon arrowroot flour
- 1/2 cup whole milk (or 3/4 cup coconut milk for dairy-free)
- 1/2 cup heavy cream (or 1/4 cup coconut cream for dairy-free)
- Pinch saffron (optional)
- 1 teaspoon Celtic sea salt
- 1/4 teaspoon freshly ground black pepper

Instructions

1. Bring a large pot of water to boil.

2. Place kale in the boiling water and continue to boil for 8 minutes.

3. Drain and squeeze excess moisture out of kale (this can be done a day or two ahead and time.

4. Just store the kale in the fridge until ready to continue with the recipe).

5. Melt the butter in a large sauté pan over medium heat.

6. Add the shallots and cook, stirring frequently until just turning brown on the edges, about 10 minutes.

7. Stir in the garlic and cook for about 30 seconds.

8. Stir in the arrowroot flour and then the milk and cream.

9. Continue to cook, stirring constantly, until the mixture begins to thicken, about 2-3 minutes.

10. Add the crumbled saffron (if desired), and then stir in the kale until it's coated with the creamy milk mixture.

11. Continue cooking until the kale is heated through.

12. Stir in the salt and pepper.

13. If the mixture is too thick, you can thin it with a little milk.

14. Taste and see if kale needs a bit more salt or pepper.

15. Serve.

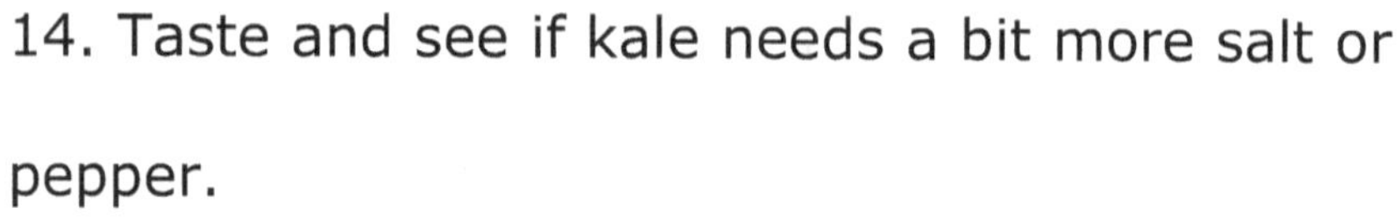

SAUSAGE, BACON AND APPLE

BREAKFAST SKILLET

Prepartion time

15 minutes

Ingredients

- 8 slices bacon, cut into small pieces

- 8 ounces sausage links, cut into small coins

- 4 apples, peeled, cored and cut into bite-size pieces

- 1 tablespoon unsalted butter (omit for dairy-free)

- 1/4 teaspoon Celtic sea salt

Instructions

1. Cook the bacon over medium heat, stirring often, until it's crispy.

2. Add the sausage to the bacon and cook for 2-3 minutes, until the sausage is just turning golden brown on the edges. (At this point, if

there's more than a tablespoon or two of fat in
the bottom of the pan, drain the pan).

3. Add the apples and cook for about 1 minute
until the apples are hot.

4. Add the butter and stir until melted.

5. Sprinkle with sea salt and serve.

www.ingramcontent.com/pod-product-compliance
Lightning Source LLC
Chambersburg PA
CBHW071910120726
48001CB00005B/1683